# The Keto Diet Cookbook

The Best Guide with Delicious Ketogenic Recipes; Many Recipes to your Satisfaction and for Good Health

## Chloe Roberts

## Disclaimer Notice:

Please note the information contained within this document is for educational and entertainment purposes only. All effort has been executed to present accurate, up to date, and reliable, complete information. No warranties of any kind are declared or implied. Readers acknowledge that the author is not engaging in the rendering of legal, financial, medical or professional advice. The content within this book has been derived from various sources. Please consult a licensed professional before attempting any techniques outlined in this book.

By reading this document, the reader agrees that under no circumstances is the author responsible for any losses, direct or indirect, which are incurred as a result of the use of information contained within this document, including, but not limited to, errors, omissions, or inaccuracies.

# Table of Content

# Introduction

Thank you for purchasing **The Keto Diet Cookbook: The Best Guide with Delicious Ketogenic Recipes; Many Recipes to your Satisfaction and for Good Health**

The ketogenic diet is a dietary regimen that drastically reduces carbohydrates, while increasing proteins and especially fats. The main purpose of this imbalance in the proportions of macronutrients in the diet is to force the body to use fats as a source of energy.

In the presence of carbohydrates, in fact, all cells use their energy to carry out their activities. But if these are reduced to a sufficiently low level they begin to use fats, all except nerve cells that do not have the ability to do so. A process called ketosis is then initiated, because it leads to the formation of molecules called ketone bodies, this time usable by the brain. Typically ketosis is achieved after a couple of days with a daily carbohydrate intake of about 20-50 grams, but these amounts can vary on an individual basis.

# BREAKFAST

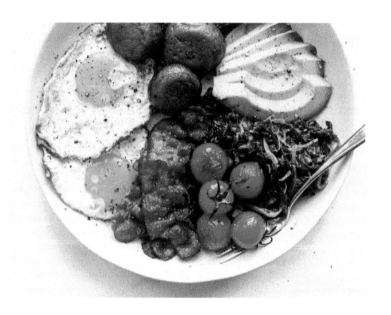

# Chocolate Chip Muffins

Preparation time: 10 minutes

Cooking time: 20 minutes

Servings: 8

Ingredients:

- ½ cup coconut flour

- ¼ tsp baking soda

- ¼ tsp salt

- 4 eggs

- 1/3 cup unsalted butter, melted

- ½ cup low-carb sweetener

- 1 tbsp vanilla extract

- 2 tbsp coconut milk

- 1/3 cup sugar-free chocolate chips

Directions:

- Preheat the oven to 350F.

- Add the coconut flour, baking soda, and salt in a bowl and blend well.

- Add the butter, eggs, sweetener, vanilla, and coconut milk to the dry ingredients and mix well. Gently stir in the chocolate chips.
- Line muffin tins and fill ¾.
- Bake for 20 minutes.
- Cool and serve.

Nutrition: Calories: 168 Fat: 13g Carb: 6g Protein: 5g

# Brownie Muffins

Preparation time: 10 minutes

Cooking time: 15 minutes

Servings: 6


Ingredients:

- ½ tsp salt

- 1 cup flaxseed meal

- ¼ cup cocoa powder

- 1 tbsp cinnamon

- ½ tbsp baking powder

- 2 tbsp coconut oil

- 1 egg

- ¼ cup sugar-free caramel syrup

- 1 tsp vanilla extract

- ½ cup pumpkin puree

- ½ cup slivered almonds

- 1 tsp apple cider vinegar

Directions:

1.     Preheat the oven to 350F.

2.     Put all everything (except the almonds) in a bowl and mix well.

3.     Place 6 paper liners in the muffin tin and add ¼-cup batter to each one.

4.     Sprinkle almonds and press gently.

5.     Bake for 15 minutes or until the top is set.

Nutrition: Calories: 183 Fat: 13g Carb: 4.4g Protein: 6.4g

# Creamy Protein Muffins

Preparation time: 5 minutes

Cooking time: 25 minutes

Servings: 12

Ingredients:

- 8 eggs

- 8 ounces cream cheese

- 2 tbsp whey protein

- 4 tbsp melted butter, cooled

Directions:

1. Heat up the oven to 350F.

2. Add melted butter and cream cheese in a bowl and mix.

3. Add whey protein and eggs into the bowl and mix until fully combined, using a hand mixer.

4. Put batter into a prepared muffin tin and transfer into the preheated oven.

5. Bake for 25 minutes.

6. Serve.

Nutrition: Calories: 165.1 Fat: 13.6g Carb: 1.5g Protein: 9.6g

# KETO BREAD

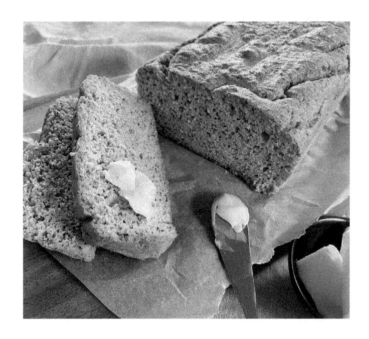

# Basic Rye Bread:

Preparation time: 2 hours

Cooking time: 3 hours

Servings: 6

Ingredients:

- 1 cup + 2 tablespoons warm water

- 2 tablespoons (40 g) molasses

- 1 tablespoon (15 ml) vegetable oil, for example, canola

- 9 g salt

- 2 cups (250 g) Bread Flour

- 187.5 g Stone Ground Whole Grain Rye Flour

- 3 tablespoons (45 g) pressed light or dull dark colored sugar

- 8 g unsweetened cocoa powder

- 3/4 teaspoon (1.5 g) caraway seeds

- 8 g Fast-Rise Yeast

Directions:

1. Spot ingredients in bread skillet as per maker's bearings. Select the entire wheat cycle with a light hull setting and begin the machine.

2.     Yield: One I-pound (455-g) portion

3.     Set machine on the mixture cycle. When the cycle is processed, structure batter into a loaf and spot in lubed 22.5 cm x 12.5 cm x 7.5-cm container.

4.     Enable the second ascent to top of container and heat in 350F stove for about 35 - 40 minutes or until moment read thermometer embedded in focus enrolls at any rate 190. Turn out to wiring rack for cooling.

Nutrition: Cal: 265, Carbs: 4 g Fiber: 12 g, Fat: 13 g, Protein: 35 g, Sugars: 1 g.

# Pita Bread

Preparation Time: 10 minutes

Cooking Time: 15 minutes

Servings: 8

Ingredients:

- 2 cups almond flour, sifted

- 1/2 cup water

- 2 Tbsp. olive oil

- Salt, to taste

- 1 tsp. black cumin

Directions:

1. Preheat the oven to 400F.

2. Combine the flour with salt. Add the water and olive oil.

3. Massage the dough and let stand for 15 minutes.

4. Shape the dough into 8 balls.

5. Put a parchment paper on the baking sheet and flatten the balls into 8 thin rounds.

6. Sprinkle black cumin.

7. Bake for 15 minutes, serve.

Nutrition: Calories: 73 Fat: 6.9g Carb: 1.6g Protein: 1.6g

# Best Keto Garlic Bread

Preparation Time: 10

Cooking Time: 15

Servings: 4

Ingredients:

- Garlic and Herb Compound Butter:

- 1/2 cup mellowed unsalted margarine (113 g/4 oz.)

- 1/2 tsp. salt (I like pink Himalayan salt)

- 1/4 tsp. ground dark pepper

- 2 tbsp. additional virgin olive oil (30 ml)

- 4 cloves garlic, squashed

- 2 tbsp. naturally slashed parsley or 2 tsp. dried parsley

- Topping:

- 1/2 cup ground Parmesan cheddar (45 g/1.6 oz.)

- 2 tbsp. crisp parsley

Directions:

1.  Set up the Keto sourdough rolls by following this formula (you can make 8 standard or 16 smaller than usual loaves). The Best Low-Carb Garlic Bread

2.      Set up the garlic margarine (or some other seasoned spread). Ensure every one of the fixings has arrived at room temperature before blending them in a medium bowl. The Best Low-Carb Garlic Bread

3.      Cut the prepared rolls down the middle and spread the enhanced margarine over every half (1-2 teaspoons for each piece). The Best Low-Carb Garlic Bread

4.      Sprinkle with ground Parmesan and spot back in the stove to fresh up for a couple of more minutes. The Best Low-Carb Garlic Bread

5.      At the point when done, expel from the stove. Alternatively, sprinkle with some olive oil and serve while still warm.

Nutrition: Calories 270, Fat 15, Fiber 3, Carbs 5, Protein 9

# Gluten-Free Brown Rice Flour Bread:

Preparation time: 2 hours

Cooking time: 3 hours

Servings: 6

Ingredients:

- 315 ml warm water

- 3 huge eggs or equal egg substitute

- 1 teaspoon (5 ml) juice vinegar

- 3 tablespoons (45 ml) vegetable oil, for example, canola oil

- 125 g unsweetened fruit purée

- 112.5 g squashed banana, or 1/2 cup (112.5 g) canned pumpkin

- 2 tablespoons (30 g) stuffed light or dull dark colored sugar

- 2 cups (250 g) Stone Ground Whole Grain Brown Rice Flour

- 1 cup (130 g) Pure Corn Starch

- 2 teaspoons (14 g) thickener

- 5 g Fast-Rise Yeast

Directions:

1. Spot water, eggs, vinegar, oil, fruit purée, and dark-colored sugar in bread dish. In a bowl, combine dark colored rice flour, corn starch, and thickener and add to skillet, alongside yeast. Begin on the battery cycle.

2. Set machine on the mixture cycle. When the cycle is processed, structure batter into a loaf and spot in lubed 22.5 cm x 12.5 cm x 7.5-cm container.

3. Enable the second ascent to top of container and heat in 350°F stove for about 35 - 40 minutes or until moment read thermometer embedded in focus enrolls at any rate 190°.

4. Yield: One I-pound (455-g) portion

Nutrition: Cal: 265, Carbs: 4 g Fiber: 12 g, Fat: 13 g, Protein: 35 g, Sugars: 1 g.

# Sourdough bread

Preparation Time: 6 minutes

Cooking Time: 15 minutes

Serving: 10

Ingredients:

- ½ cup almond flour
- ½ cup coconut flour
- ½ cup ground flaxseed
- 1/3 cup psyllium husk powder
- tsp. baking soda
- 1 tsp. Himalayan salt
- eggs
- 6 egg whites
- ¾ cup buttermilk
- ¼ cup apple cider vinegar
- ½ cup warm water

Directions:

1.     Combine the flours, flaxseed, psyllium husk, baking soda, and salt into a bowl, mix together, and set aside.

2.     Place eggs, egg whites, and buttermilk into bread machine baking pan.

3.     Add dry ingredients on top, and then pour over vinegar and warm water.

4.     Set bread machine to French setting (or a similar longer setting).

5.     Check dough during kneading process to see if more water may be needed.

6.     When the bread is done, remove bread machine pan from the bread machine.

7.     Let cool slightly before transferring to a cooling rack.

8.     The bread can be stored for up to 10 days in the fridge or for 3 months in the freezer.

Nutrition: Calories 85 Carbohydrates 4 g Fats 4 g Protein 6 g

# Toast Bread

Preparation time: 3 1/2 hours

Cooking time: 3 1/2 hours

Servings: 8

Ingredients:

* 1 1/2 teaspoons yeast

* 3 cups almond flour

* 2 tablespoons sugar

* 1 teaspoon salt

* 1 1/2 tablespoon butter

* 1 cup water

Directions

1. Pour water into the bowl; add salt, sugar, soft butter, flour, and yeast.

2. I add dried tomatoes and paprika.

3. Put it on the basic program.

4. The crust can be light or medium.

Nutrition: Carbohydrates 5 g Fats 2.7 g Protein 5.2 g Calories 203 Fiber 1 g

# Honey Whole Wheat Bread:

Preparation time: 1 hour

Cooking time: 3 hours

Servings: 5

Ingredients:

- 265 ml warm water

- 60 g nectar

- 2 g salt

- 187.5 g Stone Ground Whole Grain Whole Wheat
Graham Flour

- 187.5 g Bread Flour

- 6 g vegetable oil, for example, canola

- 6 g Fast-Rise Yeast

Directions:

1.    Spot ingredients in bread skillet as per maker's
bearings. Select entire wheat and begin the machine.

2.    Yield: 455-g loaf

3.    Set machine on the mixture cycle. When the cycle is
processed, structure batter into a loaf and spot in lubed 22.5
cm x 12.5 cm x 7.5-cm skillet.

4. Enable the second ascent to the top of dish and heat in 350F broiler for about 35 - 40 minutes or until moment read thermometer embedded in focus enlists in any event 190F.

Nutrition: Cal: 214, Carbs: 1.5 g Fiber: 8 g, Fat: 11 g, Protein: 25 g, Sugars: 1 g.

# Bread De Soul

Preparation Time: 10 minutes

Cooking time: 45 minutes

Servings: 16

Ingredients:

- 1/4 tsp. cream of tartar

- 2 1/2 tsp. baking powder

- 1tsp. xanthan gum

- 1/3 tsp. baking soda

- 1/2 tsp. salt

- 2/3 cup unflavored whey protein

- 1/4 cup olive oil

- 1/4 cup heavy whipping cream

- 2drops of sweet leaf stevia

- 2egg

- 1/4 cup butter

- 12 oz. softened cream cheese

Directions:

1. Preheat the oven to 325F.

2.	Using a bowl, microwave cream cheese and butter for 1 minute.

3.	Remove and blend well with a hand mixer.

4.	Add olive oil, eggs, heavy cream, and few drops of sweetener and blend well.

5.	Blend the dry ingredients in another bowl.

6.	Mix the wet ingredients with the dry ones and mix using a spoon. Don't use a hand blender to avoid whipping it too much.

7.	Lubricate a bread pan and pour the mixture into the pan.

8.	Bake in the oven until golden brown, about 45 minutes.

9.	Cool and serve.

Nutrition: Calories: 200 Fat: 15.2g Carb: 1.8g Protein: 10g

# Keto Pumpkin Bread Loaf

Preparation Time: 7 minutes

Cooking Time: 25 min

Serving: 14

Ingredients:

- 3 huge eggs

- ½ cup olive oil

- teaspoon vanilla concentrate

- 1/2 cups almond flour

- 1 1/2 cups erythritol

- ½ teaspoon salt

- 1 1/2 teaspoons preparing powder

- ½ teaspoon nutmeg

- 1 teaspoon ground cinnamon

- ¼ teaspoon ground ginger

- 1 cup ground zucchini

- ½ cup hacked pecans

Directions:

1. Preheat stove to 350°F. Whisk together the eggs, oil, and vanilla concentrate. Set to the side.

2.    In another bowl, combine the almond flour, erythritol, salt, heating powder, nutmeg, cinnamon, and ginger. Set to the side.

3.    Using a cheesecloth or paper towel, take the zucchini and crush out the overabundance water.

4.    Then, whisk the zucchini into the bowl with the eggs.

5.    Slowly include the dry fixings into the egg blend utilizing a hand blender until completely mixed.

6.    Lightly shower a 9x5 portion dish, and spoon in the zucchini bread blend.

7.    Then, spoon in the hacked pecans over the zucchini bread. Press pecans into the hitter utilizing a spatula.

8.    Bake for 60-70 minutes at 350°F or until the pecans on top look sautéed.

Nutrition: Cal: 70, Carbs: 3g Net Carbs: 2.5 g, Fiber: 6.5 g, Fat: 7 g, Protein: 10g, Sugars: 3 g.

# Low-Carb Cauliflower Bread

Preparation Time: 20 minutes

Cooking Time: 45 min

Serving: 8

Ingredients:

- 2 cups almond flour

- 5 eggs

- 1/4 cup psyllium husk

- 1 cup cauliflower rice

Directions

1. Preheat broiler to 350 F.

2. Line a portion skillet with material paper or coconut oil cooking shower. Put in a safe spot.

3. In an enormous bowl or nourishment processor, blend the almond flour and psyllium husk.

4. Beat in the eggs on high for as long as two minutes.

5. Blend in the cauliflower rice and mix well.

6. Empty the cauliflower blend into the portion skillet.

7. Heat for as long as 55 minutes.

Nutrition: 398 Calories; 21g Fat; 4.7g Carbs; 4.2g Protein; 0

# Rosemary & Garlic Coconut Flour Bread

Preparation Time: 20 minutes

Cooking Time: 45 min

Ingredients:

- 1/2 cup Coconut flour

- 1 sticks margarine (8 tbsp.)

- 6 enormous eggs

- 1 tsp. heating powder

- 2 tsp. Dried Rosemary

- 1/2-1 tsp. garlic powder

- 1/2 tsp. Onion powder

- 1/4 tsp. Pink Himalayan Salt

Directions:

1. Join dry fixings (coconut flour, heating powder, onion, garlic, rosemary, and salt) in a bowl and put in a safe spot.

2. Add 6 eggs to a different bowl and beat with a hand blender until you get see rises at the top.

3. Soften the stick of margarine in the microwave and gradually add it to the eggs as you beat with the hand blender.

4. When wet and dry fixings are completely consolidated in isolated dishes, gradually add the dry fixings to the wet fixings as you blend in with the hand blender.

5. Oil an 8x4 portion dish and empty the blend into it equitably.

6. Heat at 350 for 40-50 minutes (time will change contingent upon your broiler).

7. Let it rest for 10 minutes before expelling from the container. Cut up and appreciate it with spread or toasted!

Nutrition: 398 Calories; 21g Fat; 4.7g Carbs; 4.2g Protein; 0Sugars .5g

# Italian Pesto Wheat Bread:

Preparation time: 1 hour

Cooking time: 2 hours

Servings: 3

Ingredients:

- 148 ml warm water
- 14 g sugar
- 3 g salt
- 65 g arranged pesto
- 187.5 g Bread Flour
- 62.5 g Stone Ground Whole Grain Whole Wheat

Graham Flour

- 4 g Fast-Rise Yeast

Directions:

1.      Place all ingredients in a bread dish as indicated by the producer's bearings. Select essential cycles for a customary loaf or entire wheat cycle for the huge loaf and begin the machine.

2.      Yield: 455-g ordinary or 682.5-g enormous loaf

3.      Set machine on batter cycle.

4. Prepare in 350F stove for about 35 - 40 minutes or until moment read thermometer embedded in focus enlists at any rate 190F.

Nutrition: Cal: 214, Carbs: 1.5 g Fiber: 8 g, Fat: 11 g, Protein: 25 g, Sugars: 1 g.

# KETO PASTA

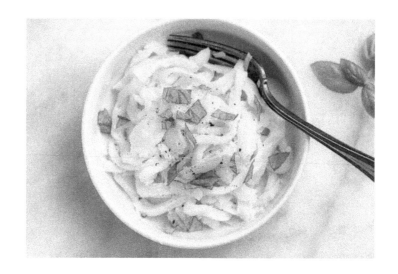

# Cauli Mac-n-Cheese

Preparation time: 10 minutes

Cooking time: 25 minutes

Servings: 3

Ingredients

- Cauliflower (1 head)

- Butter (3 tablespoons)

- Unsweetened almond milk (.25 cup)

- Heavy cream (.25 cup)

- Cheddar cheese (1 cup)

- salt and black pepper

Directions:

1. Slice the cauliflower into small florets and shred the cheese.

2. Prepare the oven to 450 Fahrenheit and cover a baking tray with a sheet of parchment paper or foil.

3. Melt 2 tbsp. of butter in a pan and toss in the florets. Give it a shake of pepper and salt.

4.      Warm up the rest of the butter, heavy cream, milk, and cheese in the microwave or double boiler. Pour the cheese over the cauliflower and serve.

Nutrition: Calories: 265 Fat: 25 g Carb: 3 g Protein: 21 g

# Edamame Kelp Noodles

Preparation time: 10 minutes

Cooking time: 30 minutes

Servings: 2

Ingredients

- Kelp noodles (1 package)

- Frozen spinach (1 cup)

- Shelled edamame (.5 cup)

- Julienned carrots (.25 cup)

- Sliced mushrooms (.25 cup)

- The Sauce:

- Sesame oil (1 tablespoon)

- Tamari (2 tablespoons)

- Ground ginger (.5 teaspoon)

- Garlic powder (.5 teaspoon)

- Sriracha (.25 teaspoon)

Directions:

1.    Soak the noodles in water. Drain well.

2.    Use the medium heat temperature setting and toss the sauce fixings in a saucepan. Add the veggies and warm.

3.      Stir in the noodles and simmer for two to three minutes. Stir before serving.

Nutrition: Calories: 365 Fat: 21 g Carb: 2 g Protein: 12 g

# Fettuccine Chicken Alfredo

Preparation time: 10 minutes

Cooking time: 45 minutes

Servings: 2

Ingredients

- Butter (2 tablespoons)

- Minced garlic cloves (2)

- Dried basil (.5 teaspoon)

- Heavy cream (.5 cup)

- Grated parmesan (4 tablespoons)

- The Chicken and Noodles:

- Chicken thighs–no bones or skin (2)

- Olive oil (1 tablespoon)

- Miracle Noodles–Fettuccine (1 bag)

- Salt and pepper (as desired)

Directions:

1.    Add the butter and cloves to a large pan to sauté for two minutes. Pour the cream into the skillet and simmer two additional minutes.

2.     Toss in one tablespoon of the parmesan at a time. Add the pepper, salt, and dried basil. Simmer for 3 to 5 minutes on the low-heat temperature setting.

3.     Use a mallet to pound the chicken (1/2-inch thickness).

4.     Warm the oil in a skillet using the medium temperature setting. Add and cook the chicken for about seven minutes on each side. Shred and set aside.

5.     Prepare the package of noodles. Rinse and boil them for two minutes in a pot of water. Combine the noodles, sauce, and shredded chicken. Cook slowly for another two minutes and serve.

Nutrition: Calories: 143 Fat: 23 g Carb: 3 g Protein: 15 g

# Stir Fry Beef Noodles

Preparation time: 10 minutes

Cooking time: 7 minutes

Servings: 3

Ingredients

- Zucchini (.5 cup)

- Baby bok choy (1 bunch)

- Broccoli florets (.25 cup)

- Flank or skirt steak (8 ounces)

- Ginger (1-inch knob)

- Avocado oil/grass-fed ghee (2 tablespoons–divided)

- Coconut aminos (2 teaspoons)

Directions:

1. Discard the end of the stem off of the bok choy. Spiralize the zucchini into 6-inch noodles. Peel and chop the ginger into thin strips. Slice the steak against the grain into thin strips.

2.     In a heated pan, add one tablespoon of oil/ghee to sear the steak using the med-high temperature setting for one to two minutes on each side.

3.     Lower the temperature to medium. Pour in the remainder of the oil, ginger, broccoli, and coconut aminos to the pan. Sauté for one minute, stirring frequently.

4.     Fold in the bok choy and continue sautéing for one more minute.

5.     Simmer to reach perfection.

Nutrition: Calories: 154 Fat: 13 g Carb: 2 g Protein: 28 g

# Tri-Color Bell Pepper Antipasto Salad With Olives And Tuna

Preparation time: 5 minutes

Cooking time: 10 minutes

Serves: 4

Ingredients:

* 2 (6-ounce) cans tuna, drained

* 1/2 cup sliced black olives

* 1/4 cup balsamic vinaigrette (see here)

* 1 green bell pepper, spiralized

* 1 yellow bell pepper, spiralized

* 1 red bell pepper, spiralized

* 1/2 cup cherry tomatoes, halved

* Salt

* Freshly ground black pepper

Directions:

1. In a large bowl, mix to combine the tuna and olives with the balsamic vinaigrette. Add the bell pepper noodles and cherry tomatoes and toss to combine. Season with salt and pepper and serve immediately.

Nutrition: Calories 270 Fat 15g, Protein 24g, Sodium 603mg,

Carbs 1g, Fiber 2g

# Sausage Goulash with Low-Carb Pasta

Preparation time: 10 minutes

Cooking time: 7 minutes

Servings: 4

Ingredients

- Shirataki ziti noodles (7-ounce package)

- Onion powder (.5 teaspoon)

- Cloves of garlic (2 minced)

- Bulk sausage (1 pound)

- Diced tomatoes (14.5-ounce can)

- Chopped celery (.25 cup)

- Stevia (1 packet)

- Salt (1 teaspoon)

- Chili powder (1 teaspoon)

Directions:

1. Drain the noodles, soak in water for 5 minutes, and drain again. Lastly, stir fry in a dry pan until the noodles feel like they're sticking to the pan.

2. Cook the sausage, onion powder, and garlic until browned.

3.     Drain the fat as needed. Add the rest of the fixings.

4.     Simmer covered for about 20 minutes. Stir often.

Nutrition: Calories: 354 Fat: 32 g Carb: 4 g Protein: 23 g

# Crispy Bacon and Sage Carbonara Noodles

Preparation time: 10 minutes

Cooking time: 25 minutes

Servings: 3

Ingredients

- Butternut squash or pumpkin (1 cup)

- Cauliflower (2 cups) Diced organic bacon (1-1.5 cups)

- noodles–zucchini noodles (3 cups)

- Turmeric (.25 to .5 teaspoon)Salt (as desired)

- Grass-fed butter or ghee (2-3 tablespoons)

- Filtered water/chicken bone broth (.25 cup)

- Fresh sage leaves (1 handful)

Directions:

1.      Steam the squash/pumpkin and cauliflower in a saucepan until softened.

2.      Dice and toss the bacon into a skillet and fry until crispy.

3.    When the bacon is ready, remove it from the skillet. Place on a paper-lined dish to drain. Leave the fat in the frying pan.

4.    Sauté the sage leaves in the bacon fat until nicely browned and crispy. Transfer the leaves into the plate with the bacon.

5.    Toss the noodles into a saucepan and steam for a few minutes.

6.    Combine the cauliflower, cooked squash/pumpkin, turmeric, butter/ghee, salt, and two tablespoons of the broth into a food processor. Pulse until smooth and creamy. Continue adding spoonsful of water/broth to reach the desired sauce consistency.

7.    When the noodles are ready, place them onto two serving platters.

8.    Pour the creamy sauce on top, adding a sprinkle of the bacon pieces and crispy sage leaves.

9.    Serve and enjoy immediately.

Nutrition: Calories: 265 Fat: 25 g Carb: 3 g Protein: 21 g

# Low carb Spaghetti & Fettuccine

Preparation time: 2 minutes

Cooking time: 3 minutes

Servings: 1

Ingredients:

- Three (3) cloves of minced garlic

- Two (2) tablespoons of butter

- Two (2) medium zucchini

- A quarter teaspoon salt to taste

- A quarter teaspoon pepper

- A quarter cup of parmesan cheese

Directions:

1. Wash your zucchini then cut it to strands using a spiralizer or vegetable peeler then set aside. If done right, your zucchini should come out like spaghetti strands. I mean, that's the point right?

2. Put a large pan on medium heat. Put the butter in to melt and then add minced garlic. Stir fry the garlic until it starts to appear translucent. If you know you have an affinity

for burning things, please be attentive so the garlic doesn't get burnt.

3.     Add your zucchini strands and stir fry for three minutes. Make sure to taste your noodle strands to check how tender they are as zucchini cooks really fast. Try not to "taste" till it finishes.

4.     Bring down the pan, add salt, pepper and parmesan cheese, stir until well combined and serve..

Nutrition: Calories: 100 Total Fat: 4g Carbs: 4g Protein: 4g

# Baked Zucchini Noodles with Feta

Preparation time: 10 minutes

Cooking time: 25 minutes

Servings: 3

Ingredients

- Spiralized zucchini (2)

- Quartered plum tomato (1)

- Feta cheese (8 cubes)

- Pepper and salt (1 teaspoon of each)

- Olive oil (1 tbsp.)

Directions:

1.      Lightly grease a roasting pan with a spritz of cooking oil.

2.      Set the oven temperature at 375 Fahrenheit.

3.      Slice the noodles with a spiralizer, and add the olive oil, tomatoes, pepper, and salt.

4.      Bake the noodle dish for 10 to 15 minutes. Transfer

from the oven and add the cheese cubes, tossing to combine.

Serve.

Nutrition: Calories: 354 Fat: 32 g Carb: 5 g Protein: 19g

# Shrimp Pad Thai and Shirataki Noodles

Preparation time: 10 minutes

Cooking time: 7 minutes

Servings: 3

Ingredients

- Shirataki fettuccini noodles (2 packs–7 ounces each)

- Medium-sized wild-caught shrimp (18)

- Pastured eggs (2)

- Brain Octane Oil–divided (1.5 tablespoons)

- Coconut aminos (2 tablespoons)

- Lime (1 juiced and divided)

- Cashew butter (1 teaspoon)

- Garlic (1 clove)

- Crushed red pepper (.25 teaspoon)

- Cilantro (.25 cup)

- Green onions (2)

- Sea salt

- Optional for the Garnish: Cashews (4 crushed)

Directions:

1.     Finely mince the garlic and onions.

2.    Prepare the shirataki noodles using the package instructions (rinsing for 15 seconds, boiling for 2 minutes in a pot of water, and draining the noodles. Place them in a dry skillet without oil using the medium heat and "dry roast" them for one minute). Set aside for now.

3.    Combine the cashew butter, 3/4 of a tablespoon of the Brain Octane Oil, garlic, coconut aminos, half of the lime juice, and crushed red pepper in a small mixing container. Set aside.

4.    Prepare a large skillet (medium heat). Stir in the last 3/4 tablespoon of oil, shrimp, and a pinch of sea salt. Simmer for about 1.5-2 minutes on each side.

5.    Whisk the eggs and spread into the skillet to the side of the shrimp. Cook the eggs to a soft scramble (1 minute).

6.    Add the sauce mixture, noodles, cilantro, and green onions. Toss well. Heat until warmed.

7.    To finish, drizzle the rest of the lime juice over the skillet, and adjust seasonings as desired.

8.    Garnish with crushed cashews before serving.

Nutrition: Calories: 354 Fat: 32 g Carb: 4 g Protein: 23 g

# Thai-Inspired Peanut Red Curry Vegan Bowl

Preparation time: 10 minutes

Cooking time: 7 minutes

Servings: 3

Ingredients

- Sesame oil (1 teaspoon)

- Shirataki noodles (8-ounce package)

- Unsweetened peanut butter (2 tablespoons)

- Low-sodium tamari (2 teaspoons)

- Thai red curry paste (2-3 teaspoons)

- Grated ginger (.25 teaspoon)

- Fresh edamame (.25 cup)

- Fresh lime juice (1 teaspoon)

Directions:

1.      Thoroughly rinse and drain the noodles and add to a frying pan using the medium-low temperature setting. Cook until the noodles are mostly dry.

2.      Stir in the curry paste, tamari, peanut butter, sesame oil, grated ginger, and bell peppers. Stir until the sauce forms, and everything is evenly coated.

3.      Simmer for about three to five more minutes or until the peppers soften, and everything is heated.

4.      Transfer the hot curry to a bowl and top with edamame and other desired toppings.

Nutrition: Calories: 324 Fat,: 16 g Carb1 2 g Protein: 13 g

# Keto Japanese Seafood Pasta

Preparation time: 5 minutes

Cooking time: 10 minutes

Servings: 2

Ingredients:

- Two (2) cloves of garlic

- Three (3) tablespoons of Heavy cream

- Half an onion(diced)

- Half a cup of Clam juice

- A teaspoon of soy sauce

- A tablespoon of salted butter

- A pack of Shirataki noodles

- A quarter teaspoon of black pepper

- A tablespoon of Kewpie mayo

- Two (2) tablespoons of white wine

- Frozen seafood mix (preferably shrimp, clams and bay scallops)

Directions:

1. If your seafood mix is frozen, thaw it until fully melted.

2. Boil a water.

3.     Strain the shirataki noodles to get rid of pre-packed liquid.

4.     Run the noodles under cold water, put in a bowl then set aside.

5.     Dice the onions and garlic then set aside.

6.     Put soy sauce, kewpie mayo, and heavy cream  into a small bowl then mix until fully combined then set aside.

7.     Attach in the shirataki noodles, and cook for 2-3 minutes (this is mostly to remove the taste of the pre-packed liquid from the noodles)

8.     Strain the noodles and set aside.

9.     Fry onions until it starts to turn brown.

10.    Add white wine, seafood mix, clam juice and garlic and cook, stirring until seafood gets completely cooked through and the liquid in the pan dries up.

11.    Pour in the sauce from step 5 and reduce the heat to low. Stir the mixture until full combined  and let cook for another minute.

12.    Pour the sauce over the shirataki noodles and enjoy!

Nutrition: Calories: 325 Total Fat: 11g Carbs: 4g Protein: 14g

# KETO CHAFFLE

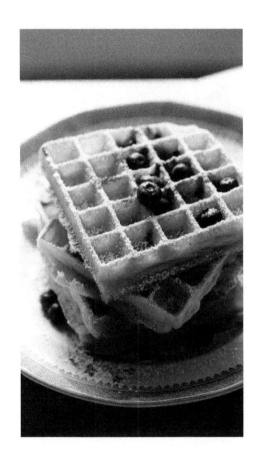

# Chicken Chickpea Chaffles

Preparation Time: 5 minutes

Cooking Time: 10 minutes

Servings: 2

Ingredients:

- Provolone  cheese (shredded) – 1 cup

- Eggs – 2

- Butter head Lettuce (optional) – 2 leaves

- Ketchup (sugar free)  – 2 tablespoons

- Soy sauce – 1 tablespoon

- Worcestershire/Worcester sauce – 2 tablespoons

- Monk fruit/swerve – 1 teaspoon

- Chicken thigh (boneless) – 2 pieces

- Chickpea flour – 3/4 cup

- Salt (as desired)

- Eggs – 1

- Black pepper – (as desired)

- Vegetable cooking oil – 2 cups

- Pork rinds – 3 oz

- Salt – 1 tablespoon

- Water – 2 cups

Directions:

1. Boil chicken for 30 min then pat it dry

2. Add black pepper and salt to the chicken

3. Mix soy sauce, Worcestershire sauce , ketchup and Swerve/Monkfruit in one bowl then set aside

4. Grind pork rinds into fine crumbs

5. In separate bowls, add the Chickpea flour, beaten eggs and the crushed pork then coat your chicken pieces using these ingredients in their listed order

6. Fry coated chicken till golden brown

7. Pre-heat and grease waffle maker

8. Mix eggs and Provolone cheese together in a bowl

9. Pour into waffle maker and cook till crunchy

10. Wash and dry green lettuces

11. Spread previously prepared sauces on one chaffle, place some lettuce, one chicken katsu then add one more chaffle

Nutrition: Calories: 125 Fat: 7g Carb: 1 g Protein: 5g

# Bacon Provolone Chaffles

Preparation Time: 5 minutes

Cooking Time: 15 minutes

Servings: 2

Ingredients:

- Provolone cheese (shredded) – 1 cup

- Eggs – 2

- Green onion (diced) – 1 tbsp

- Italian seasoning – 1/2 teaspoon

- Bacon – 4 strips

- Tomato (sliced) - 1

- (c) Butter head lettuce  – 2 leaves

- Mayo – 2 tablespoons

Directions:

1. Pre-heat and grease waffle maker

2. Mix all ingredients in one bowl

3. Pour mixture onto waffle plate and spread evenly

4. Cook till crunchy then leave to cool for a minute

5. Serve with butter head lettuce, tomato and mayo

Nutrition: Calories 115 Fat 7.3g Protein 1.4g Carbs: 4g

# Crunchy Provolone Cheese Chaffles

Preparation Time: 5 minutes

Cooking Time: 5 minutes

Servings: 2

Ingredients:

- Provolone Cheese – 1/2 cup

- Eggs – 1

- Bread crumbs – 1/2 cup

- Pickle juice – 1 tablespoon

- Pickle slices – 8

Directions:

1. Pre-heat waffle iron

2. Mix ingredients together and pour thin layer onto waffle iron

3. Add drained pickle slices

4. Top with remaining mixture and cook till crisp

Nutrition: Calories 252 Total Fat 17.3 g Total Carbs 3.2 g Sugar 0.3 g Fiber 1.4 g Protein 5.2 g

# Pancetta Bite Chaffles

Preparation Time: 12 minutes

Cooking Time: 30 minutes

Servings: 4

Ingredients:

- Pancetta bites (as desired)
- Cheddar cheese – 1 1/2 cups

Directions:

1. Pre-heat waffle iron
2. Mix all ingredients in one bowl
3. Lightly grease waffle iron
4. Pour mixture and cook till crisp

Nutrition: Calories: 321 Fat: 3 g Carb: 3 g Protein: 15 g

# Pecorino Romano. Chaffles

Preparation Time: 5 minutes

Cooking Time: 5 minutes

Servings: 2

Ingredients:

- Cheddar – 1/3 cup

- Pecorino Romano – 1/3 cup

- Eggs – 1

- Baking powder – 1/4 teaspoon

- Flaxseed (ground) – 1 teaspoon

- Olive (sliced) – 6 to 8

Directions:

1. Add cheddar cheese, flaxseed, egg and baking powder in a bowl and mix

2. Shred half Pecorino Romano cheese on waffle iron and lightly grease plate

3. Pour mixture and top with olives and remaining Pecorino Romano cheese

4. Cook till crisp

Nutrition: Calories 252 Total Fat 17.3 g Total Carbs 3.2 g Sugar 0.3 g  Fiber 1.4 g Protein 5.2 g

# Okra-Cheddar Chaffles

Preparation Time: 5 minutes

Cooking Time: 15 minutes

Servings: 6

Ingredients:

- Okra – 1 medium

- Eggs – 1

- Cheddar cheese – 1 1/2 cups

Directions:

1. Boil Okra for 15 min then blend

2. Preheat waffle iron

3. Mix listed ingredients in one bowl

4. Grease waffle iron, pour mixture and cook till crisp

Nutrition: Calories 136 Total Fat 10.7 g Total Carbs 1.2 g Sugar 1.4 g  Fiber 0.2 g Protein 0.9

# MAIN, SIDE & VEGETABLE

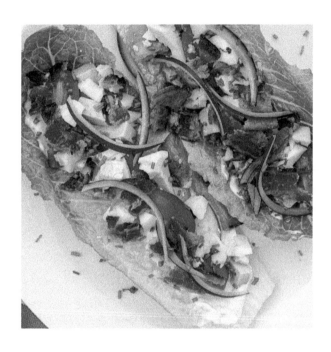

# Spicy Pork Chops

Preparation time: 4 hours and 10 minutes

Cooking time: 15 minutes

Servings: 2

Ingredients:

- ¼ cup lime juice 2 pork rib chops
- 1/2 tablespoon coconut oil, melted
- 1/2 garlic cloves, peeled and minced
- 1/2 tablespoon chili powder
- 1/2 teaspoon ground cinnamon
- teaspoon cumin
- Salt and pepper to taste
- 1/4 teaspoon hot pepper sauce
- Mango, sliced

Directions:

1. Take a bowl and mix in lime juice, oil, garlic, cumin, cinnamon, chili powder, salt, pepper, hot pepper sauce. Whisk well.

2.	Add pork chops and toss. Keep it on the side, and let it refrigerate for 4 hours.

3.	Preheat your grill to medium and transfer pork chops to the preheated grill. Grill for 7 minutes, flip and cook for 7 minutes more.

4.	Divide between serving platters and serve with mango slices. Enjoy!

Nutrition: Calories: 200 Fat: 8g Carbohydrates: 3g Protein: 26g Fiber: 1g  Net Carbohydrates: 2g

# Appealing Broccoli Mash

Preparation Time: 15 minutes

Cooking Time: 5 minutes

Servings: 6

Ingredients:

- 16 oz. broccoli florets
- C. water
- tsp. fresh lemon juice
- tsp. butter, softened
- 1 tsp. garlic, minced
- Salt and freshly ground black pepper, to taste

Directions:

1. In a medium pan, add the broccoli and water over medium heat and cook for about 5 minutes.

2. Drain the broccoli well and transfer into a large bowl

3. In the bowl of broccoli, add the lemon juice, butter, and garlic and with an immersion blender blend until smooth.

4. Season with salt and black pepper and serve.

Nutrition: Calories 32; Carbohydrates: 5.1g; Protein: 2g; Fat: 0.9g; Sugar: 1.3g; Sodium: 160mg; Fiber: 2g

# Eggs with Greens

Preparation time: 5 minutes

Cooking time: 10 minutes

Servings: 2

Ingredients:

*   3 tbsp chopped parsley
*   3 tbsp chopped cilantro
*   ¼ tsp cayenne pepper
*   2 eggs
*   tbsp butter, unsalted
*   Seasoning:
*   ¼ tsp salt
*   1/8 tsp ground black pepper

Directions:

1.   Take a medium skillet pan, place it over medium-low heat, add butter and wait until it melts.

2.   Then add parsley and cilantro, season with salt and black pepper, stir until mixed and cook for 1 minute.

3.    Make two space in the pan, crack an egg into each space, and then sprinkle with cayenne pepper, cover the pan with the lid and cook for 2 to 3 minutes until egg yolks have set.

4.    Serve.

Nutrition: 135 Calories; 11.1 g Fats; 7.2 g Protein; 0.2 g Net Carb; 0.5 g Fiber;

# Zesty Brussels Sprout

Preparation Time: 15 minutes

Cooking Time: 15 minutes

Servings: 2


Ingredients:

* ½ lb. fresh Brussels sprouts, trimmed and halved

* 2 tbsp. olive oil

* 2 small garlic cloves, minced

* ½ tsp. red pepper flakes, crushed

* Salt and freshly ground black pepper, to taste

* tbsp. fresh lemon juice

* tsp. fresh lemon zest, grated finely


Directions:

1. Arrange a steamer basket over a large pan of the boiling water.

2. Place the asparagus into the steamer basket and steam, covered for about 6-8 minutes.

3. Remove from the heat and drain the asparagus well.

4.     In a large skillet, heat the oil over medium heat and sauté the garlic and red pepper flakes for about 1 minute.

5.     Stir in the Brussels sprouts, salt and black pepper and sauté for about 4-5 minutes.

6.     Stir in the lemon juice and sauté for about 1 minute more.

7.     Remove from the heat and serve hot with the garnishing of the lemon zest.

Nutrition: Calories: 116; Carbohydrates: 11g; Protein: 4.1g; Fat: 7.5g; Sugar: 2.5g; Sodium: 102mg; Fiber: 4.4g

# Pasta Orecchiette with Broccoli & Tofu

Preparation Time: 10 minutes

Cooking Time: 15 minutes

Servings: 4

Ingredients:

- (9 oz.) pack orecchiette

- 16 oz. broccoli, roughly chopped

- garlic cloves

- tbsp. olive oil

- tbsp. grated tofu

- Salt and black pepper to taste

Directions:

1. Place the orecchiette and broccoli in your instant pot. Cover with water and seal the lid. Cook on High Pressure for 10 minutes. Do a quick release.

2. Drain the broccoli and orecchiette. Set aside. Heat the olive oil on Sauté mode. Stir-fry garlic for 2 minutes. Stir in broccoli, orecchiette, salt, and pepper. Cook for 2 more minutes. Press Cancel and Stir in grated tofu, to serve.

Nutrition: Calories: 192 kcal Protein: 7.08 g Fat: 12.6 g

Carbohydrates: 16.93 g

# Fried Eggs with Kale and Bacon

Preparation time: 5 minutes

Cooking time: 15 minutes

Servings: 2

Ingredients:

- 4 slices of turkey bacon, chopped
- bunch of kale, chopped
- oz butter, unsalted
- eggs
- 2 tbsp chopped walnuts
- Seasoning:
- 1/3 tsp salt
- 1/3 tsp ground black pepper

Directions:

1. Take a frying pan, place it over medium heat, add two-third of the butter in it, let it melt, then add kale, switch heat to medium-high level and cook for 4 to 5 minutes until edges have turned golden brown.

2.     When done, transfer kale to a plate, set aside until required, add bacon into the pan and cook for 4 minutes until crispy.

3.     Return kale into the pan, add nuts, stir until mixed and cook for 2 minutes until thoroughly warmed.

4.     Transfer kale into the bowl, add remaining butter into the pan, crack eggs into the pan and fry them for 2 to 3 minutes until cooked to the desired level.

5.     Distribute kale between two plates, add fried eggs on the side, sprinkle with salt and black pepper, and then serve.

Nutrition: 525 Calories; 50 g Fats; 14.4 g Protein; 1.1 g Net Carb; 2.8 g Fiber;

# Stuffed Chicken Breasts

Preparation time: 30 minutes

Cooking time: 30 minutes

Servings:4

Ingredients:

- tablespoon butter
- ¼ cup chopped sweet onion
- ½ cup goat cheese, at room temperature
- ¼ cup Kalamata olives, chopped
- ¼ cup chopped roasted red pepper
- tablespoons chopped fresh basil
- (5-ounce) chicken breasts, skin-on
- 2 tablespoons extra-virgin olive oil

Directions:

1. Preheat the oven to 400°F.

2. In a small skillet over medium heat, melt the butter and add the onion. Sauté until tender, about 3 minutes.

3. Transfer the onion to a medium bowl and add the cheese, olives, red pepper, and basil. Stir until well blended, then refrigerate for about 30 minutes.

4.     Cut horizontal pockets into each chicken breast, and stuff them evenly with the filling. Secure the two sides of each breast with toothpicks.

5.     Place a large ovenproof skillet over medium-high heat and add the olive oil.

6.     Brown the chicken on both sides, about 10 minutes in total.

7.     Place the skillet in the oven and roast until the chicken is just cooked through, about 15 minutes. Remove the toothpicks and serve.

Nutrition: Calories: 389 Fat: 30g Protein: 25g Carbohydrates: 3g Fiber: 0g

# Spicy Chaffle with Jalapeno

Preparation time: 5 minutes

Cooking time: 10 minutes;

Servings: 2

Ingredients:

- 2 tsp coconut flour
- ½ tbsp chopped jalapeno pepper
- 2 tsp cream cheese
- egg
- oz shredded mozzarella cheese
- Seasoning:
- ¼ tsp salt
- 1/8 tsp ground black pepper

Directions:

1. Switch on a mini waffle maker and let it preheat for 5 minutes.

2. Meanwhile, take a medium bowl, place all the ingredients in it and then mix by using an immersion blender until smooth.

3. Ladle the batter evenly into the waffle maker, shut with lid, and let it cook for 3 to 4 minutes until firm and golden brown.

4. Serve.

Nutrition: 153 Calories; 10.7 g Fats; 11.1 g Protein; 1 g Net Carb; 1 g Fiber;

# SOUP AND STEWS

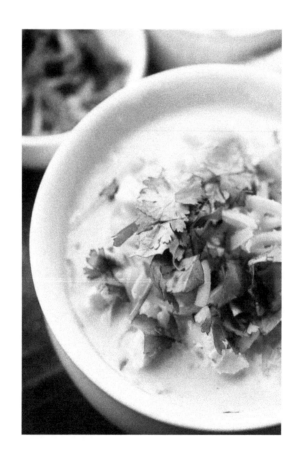

# Vegetarian Garlic, Tomato & Onion Soup

Preparation time: 15 minutes

Cooking time: 30 minutes

Servings: 6

Ingredients:

* 6 cups vegetable broth

* ½ cup full-fat unsweetened coconut milk

* 1½ cups canned diced tomatoes

* yellow onion, chopped

* cloves garlic, chopped

* teaspoon Italian seasoning

* bay leaf

* Pinch of salt & pepper, to taste

* Fresh basil, for serving

Directions:

1. Add all the ingredients minus the coconut milk and fresh basil to a stockpot over medium heat and bring to a boil. Reduce to a simmer and cook for 30 minutes.

2.      Remove the bay leaf, and then use an immersion blender to blend the soup until smooth. Stir in the coconut milk.

3.      Garnish with fresh basil and serve.

Nutrition: Calories: 104 Carbs: 6g Fiber: 1g Net Carbs: 5g Fat: 7g Protein: 6g

# Hot Sauce

Preparation Time: 15 minutes

Cooking Time: 15 minutes

Servings: 40

Ingredients:

- tablespoon olive oil

- cup carrot, peeled and chopped

- ½ cup yellow onion, chopped

- 5 garlic cloves, minced

- 6 habanero peppers, stemmed

- tomato, chopped

- 1 tablespoon fresh lemon zest

- ¼ cup fresh lemon juice

- ¼ cup balsamic vinegar

- ¼ cup water

- Salt and ground black pepper, as required

Directions:

1.     Heat the oil in a huge pan over medium heat and cook the carrot, onion, and garlic for about 8-10 minutes, stirring frequently.

2.    Remove the pan from heat and let it cool slightly.

3.    Place the onion mixture and remaining ingredients in a food processor and pulse until smooth.

4.    Return the mixture into the same pan over medium-low heat and simmer for about 3-5 minutes, stirring occasionally.

5.    Remove the pan from heat and let it cool completely.

6.    You can preserve this sauce in the refrigerator by placing it into an airtight container.

Nutrition: Calories: 9 Net Carbs: 1g Carbohydrate: 1.3g Fiber: 0.3g Protein: 0.2g Fat: 0.4g Sugar: 0.7g Sodium: 7mg

# Carrot, Ginger & Turmeric Soup

Preparation time: 15 minutes

Cooking time: 40 minutes

Servings: 8

Ingredients:

- 6 cups vegetable broth
- ¼ cup full-fat unsweetened coconut milk
- ¾ pound carrots, peeled and chopped
- 2 teaspoons grated ginger
- teaspoon ground turmeric
- sweet yellow onion, chopped
- cloves garlic, chopped
- Pinch of sea salt & pepper, to taste

Directions:

1. Add all the ingredients minus the coconut milk to a stockpot over medium heat and bring to a boil. Reduce to a simmer and cook for 40 minutes or until the carrots are tender.

2. Use an immersion blender and blend the soup until smooth. Stir in the coconut milk.

3.     Enjoy right away and freeze any leftovers.

Nutrition: Calories: 73 Carbs: 7g Fiber: 2g Net Carbs: 5g Fat: 3g Protein: 4g

# Green Jalapeno Sauce

Preparation Time: 5 minutes

Cooking Time: 0 minutes

Servings: 1

Ingredients:

- ½ avocado

- large jalapeno

- cup fresh cilantro

- tablespoons extra virgin olive oil

- tablespoons water

- Water

- ½ teaspoon salt

Directions:

1. Add all ingredients in a blender.

2. Blend until smooth and creamy.

3. Serve and enjoy.

Nutrition: Calories: 407 Fat: 42g Carbs: 10g Protein: 2.4g

# Beef Cabbage Soup

Preparation Time: 10 minutes

Cooking Time: 20 minutes

Servings: 8

Ingredients:

- 2 tbsp. Olive oil

- large Onion

- lb. Ribeye fillet steak

- stalk Celery

- large Carrots

- 1 small Green cabbage

- cloves Garlic

- 6 cups Beef stock/broth

- tbsp. + more for serving Fresh chopped parsley

- tsp. Dried thyme /rosemary/ basil & oregano

- tsp. Onion/garlic powder

- Freshly-cracked black pepper & salt (as desired)

Directions:

1.   Mince the garlic and chop the onion, celery, and carrots. Chop the cabbage into bite-sized chunks. Trim the steak of all visible fat. Chop into one-inch chunks.

2.   Warm oil in a large pot using the medium heat temperature setting.

3.   Toss in the cut meat. Sear until browned. Toss in the onions and sauté until transparent (3-4 min.).

4.   Toss in the celery and carrots, mixing well for about 3-4 minutes.

5.   Fold in the cabbage and sauté an additional five minutes. Toss in the garlic, and sauté for another minute, mixing all fixings through.

6.   in the stock/broth, dried herbs, parsley, and onion or garlic powder, mixing well. Simmer and reduce the heat to med-low. Cover with a top.

7.   Simmer until the cabbage and carrots are softened (10 to 15 min.). Toss the salt, pepper, and extra dried herbs, as desired. Serve warm.

Nutrition: Calories: 177 Net Carbs: 4 g Total Fat Content: 11 g Protein: 12 g

# DESSERT

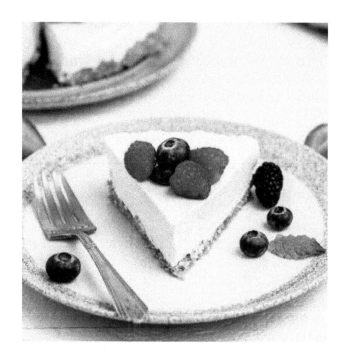

# Pistachio Cookies

Preparation Time: 10 minutes

Cooking Time: 25 minutes

Servings: 8

Ingredients:

- 3/4 cup (4 oz.) shelled pistachio nuts

- 2 tsp. + 1 cup stevia granulated sweetener

- 1 2/3 cup almond meal or almond flour

- 2 eggs, beaten well

Directions:

1. Add pistachio and stevia to a food processor and pulse until finely ground.

2. Toss pistachio mixture with almond meal or flour in a bowl.

3. Add eggs and whisk well until combined.

4. Refrigerate this mixture for 8 hours or overnight.

5. Let your oven preheat at 325 degrees F.

6. Layer a cookie sheet with wax paper then use a scoop or spoon to add the cookie dough to the sheet scoop by scoop.

7. Bake them for 25 minutes until lightly brown.

8.     Allow them to cool then serve.

Nutrition: Calories 174 Total Fat 12.3 G Carbs 4.5 G Fiber 0.6 G Sugar 1.9 G  Protein 12 G

# Almond Butter Cookies

Preparation Time: 5 minutes

Cooking Time: 12 minutes

Servings: 14

Ingredients:

- 1 cup smooth almond butter

- 4 tbsp unsweetened cocoa powder

- 1/2 cup granulated erythritol sweetener

- 1/4 cup sugar-free chocolate chips

- 1 large egg

- 3 tbsp almond milk unsweetened, if needed

Directions:

1. Preheat your oven at 350 degrees F.

2. Whisk almond butter together with granulated sweetener, egg, and cocoa powder in a bowl with a fork. Add 3 tbsp almond milk if the mixture is too crumbly.

3. Fold in chocolate chips then make 6-centimeterround cookie balls out of it.

4. Place the balls on a baking sheet lined with parchment paper.

5.     Bake them for 12 minutes then allow them to cool.

6.     Enjoy.

Nutrition: Calories 77.8 Total Fat 7.13 g Total Carbs 0.8 g Sugar 0.2 g Fiber 0.3 g Protein 2.3 g

# Macadamia Nut Cookies

Preparation Time: 10 minutes

Cooking Time: 15 minutes

Servings: 12

Ingredients:

- 1/2 cup butter, melted
- 2 tbsp almond butter
- 1 egg
- 1 1/2 cup almond flour
- 2 tbsp unsweetened cocoa powder
- 1/2 cup granulated erythritol sweetener
- 1 tsp vanilla extract
- 1/2 tsp baking soda
- 1/4 cup chopped macadamia nuts
- Pinch of salt

Directions:

1. Preheat your oven to 350 degrees F.

2.     Whisk all the ingredients well in a bowl with a fork until smooth.

3.     Layer a cookie sheet with wax paper and drop the dough onto it scoop by scoop.

4.     Flatten each scoop into 1.5-inch wide round.

5.     Bake them for 15 minutes then allow them to cool.

6.     Enjoy.

Nutrition: Calories 114 Total Fat 9.6 g Total Carbs 3.1 g Sugar 1.4 g Fiber 1.5 g Protein 3.5 g

# Stuffed Oreo Cookies

Preparation Time: 5 minutes

Cooking Time: 12 minutes

Servings: 8

Ingredients:

- 1 1/3 cup almond flour

- 6 tbsp cocoa powder

- 2 tbsp black cocoa powder

- 3/4 tsp kosher salt

- 1/2 tsp xanthan gum

- 1/2 tsp baking soda

- 1/4 tsp espresso powder

- 5 1/2 tbsp butter

- 8 tbsp erythritol

- 1 egg

- For Vanilla Cream Filling

- 4 tbsp grass-fed butter

- 1 tbsp coconut oil

- 1 1/2 tsp vanilla extract

- Pinch kosher salt

- 1/2 - 1 cup Swerve confectioner sugar substitute

Directions:

1. Whisk almond flour, salt, both cocoa powders, xanthan gum, baking soda, and espresso powder in a suitable bowl.

2. Beat butter well in a large bowl with a hand mixer for 2 minutes.

3. Whisk in sweetener and continue beating for 5 minutes then add the egg.

4. Beat well then add the flour mixture. Mix well until fully incorporated.

5. Wrap the cookie dough with plastic wrap and refrigerate for 1 hour.

6. Meanwhile, preheat your oven to 350 degrees F and layer a baking sheet with wax paper.

7. Place the dough in between two sheets of parchment paper.

8. Roll the dough out into a 1/8-inch thick sheet.

9. Cut 1 3/4 inch round cookies out of this sheet and reroll the dough to cut more cookies.

10. Spread these cookies on the baking sheet and freeze for 15 minutes.

11. Bake these cookies for 12 minutes then allow them to cool on a wire rack.

12. Beat butter with coconut oil in a bowl with an electric mixer.

13. Stir in vanilla extract, powdered sweetener to taste, and a pinch of salt.

14. Mix well then transfer it to a piping bag.

15. Place half of the cookies on a cookie sheet and top them with the cream filling.

16. Place the remaining half of the cookies over the filling to cover it.

17. Refrigerate for 15 minutes then serve.

Nutrition: Calories 215 Total Fat 20 g Total Carbs 3 g Sugar 1 g Fiber 6 g Protein 5 g

# Vanilla Berry Meringues

Preparation Time: 15 minutes

Cooking Time: 1 hour and 45 minutes

Servings: 10

Ingredients:

- teaspoon vanilla extract
- tablespoons freeze-dried mixed berries, crushed
- large egg whites, at room temperature
- 1/3 cup Erythritol
- teaspoon lemon rind

Directions:

1. In a mixing bowl, stir the egg whites until foamy. Add in vanilla extract, lemon rind, and Erythritol; continue to mix, using an electric mixer until stiff and glossy.

2. Add the crushed berries and mix again until well combined. Use two teaspoons to spoon the meringue onto parchment-lined cookie sheets.

3. Bake at 220 degrees F for about 1 hour 45 minutes.

Nutrition: 51 Calories 0g Fat 4g Carbs 12g Protein 0.1g Fiber

# Fudgy Brownie Cookies

Preparation Time: 10 minutes

Cooking Time: 12 minutes

Servings: 12

Ingredients:

- 2 tbsp. butter, softened
- 1 egg, room temperature
- 1 tbsp. Truvia
- 1/4 cup Swerve
- 1/8 tsp. blackstrap molasses
- 1 tbsp. VitaFiber syrup
- 1 tsp. vanilla extract
- 6 tbsp. sugar-free chocolate chips
- 1 tsp. butter
- 6 tbsp. almond flour
- 1 tbsp. cocoa powder
- 1/8 tsp. baking powder
- 1/8 tsp. salt
- 1/4 tsp. xanthan gum
- 1/4 cup chopped pecans

- 1 tbsp. sugar-free chocolate chips

Directions:

1. Beat egg with 2 tablespoons butter, VitaFiber, sweeteners, and vanilla in a bowl with a hand mixer.

2. Melt 1/2 of a tablespoon of the chocolate chips with 1 teaspoon of butter in a bowl by heating them in the microwave for 30 seconds then stir well.

3. Add this mixture to the first butter mixture and mix well until smooth.

4. Stir in all the dry ingredients and mix until smooth.

5. Fold in remaining chocolate chips and pecans.

6. Place this batter in the freezer for 8 minutes.

7. Let your oven preheat at 350 degrees F.

8. Grease a baking sheet and drop batter scoop by scoop onto it to form small cookies.

9. Flatten the cookies lightly then bake for 10 minutes.

10. Allow the cookies to cool for about 15 minutes then serve.

Nutrition: Calories 288 Total Fat 25.3 g Total Carbs 3.6 g Sugar 0.1 g Fiber 3.8 g Protein 7.6 g

Lightning Source UK Ltd.
Milton Keynes UK
UKHW020651210521
384114UK00001B/73